I0448012

Homemade Body Scrubs

Simple Recipes for Beautiful and Healthy Skin

Beth McRoberts

http://www.bethmcrobertsbooks.com

All Rights Reserved. No part of this publication may be reproduced in any form or by any means, including scanning, photocopying, or otherwise without prior written permission of the copyright holder. Copyright © 2014

Table of Contents

Don't Make These 9 Exfoliation Mistakes

Conclusion

Preface

No one enjoys itchy, dull skin. If you aren't exfoliating on a regular basis, you probably have this problem on at least one part of your body.

Our bodies are designed to shed the older, outer layers of skin regularly. Unfortunately, that skin doesn't just fall off all in one chunk. In fact, if you don't exfoliate, the top layer of your skin is probably made up of dead skin cells that are around a month old.

These dead skin cells not only make your body's surface look dull, they can also block pores. Oil and toxins build up in these blocked pores and cause breakouts. These can occur anywhere on your body, but are most likely on your face, back, arms and chest.

Exfoliation takes care of all these issues for you. Body scrubs consist of several ingredients, one or more of which is rough to help remove the layer of dead skin over your entire body. Exfoliating scrubs help get rid of the dull surface layer of skin and give you a glowing appearance.

When you exfoliate regularly, you'll enjoy smooth, healthy skin over your entire body. Eliminating dead cells also keeps itching at bay and will give you a more radiant glow.

While you can buy scrubs in the store and online, these are usually packed with chemicals and all sorts of harsh ingredients that you definitely don't want on your skin. Purchased scrubs are also extremely pricey for what they offer. Even if you find a product that is all natural, it will take a big bite out of your wallet.

It is surprisingly easy to mix up your own body scrubs with all natural and fresh ingredients. Every scrub you make can be tailored to your individual needs. If you need a little pick-me-up, try a peppermint sugar scrub. For a soothing, moisturizing option, you can add coconut oil, shea butter or any number of hydrating ingredients . . . most of which are in your pantry already!

This book is packed with incredibly simple recipes that absolutely anyone can make. You probably have everything necessary to create one right now. The recipes given here include energy boosting ones and moisturizing cleansers, so there's something for everyone.

5 Ways Store-bought Scrubs Are Destroying Your Body and Your World

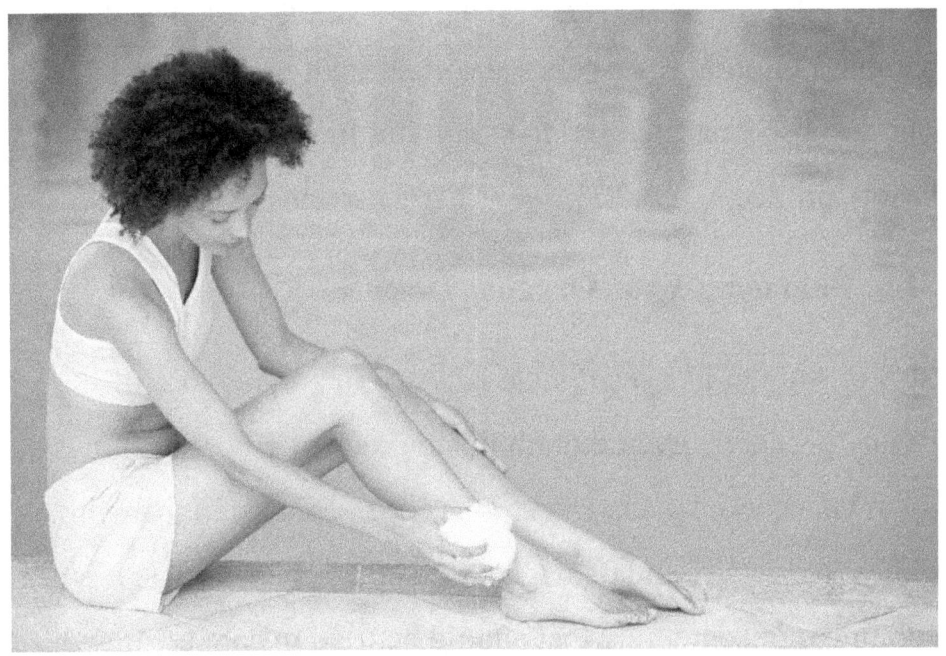

Chances are, you have at least one body scrub in your bathroom. Have you ever stopped to look at the ingredients in your lotions and body scrubs? You might be surprised at what you find.

You wouldn't eat food that was packed with chemicals that are known to be dangerous, so why would you apply those same chemicals to your skin? Unfortunately, many of the products used by women around the world are full of nasty chemicals that should never come in contact with your skin.

Parabens Increase Breast Cancer Risk

Did you know that some skin products can actually increase your chances of getting breast cancer? If your scrub has parabens in it, they are being absorbed right through your skin. These substances are used to stop mold from growing on your beauty products, but the price is hardly worth it.

SLS: Damaging Your Organs

SLS or sodium lauryl sulphate is found in around 90% of beauty products. Even though this ingredient probably shows up in your lotions and scrubs, it has been connected to health issues like cancer and damage to the kidneys and lungs. It is certainly not something that should be used in connection with your body.

Preserve Your Face with Formaldehyde

Remember that sickly sweet smell in Biology class when you had to dissect an animal? That smell was formaldehyde, a preservative chemical. It's known to be a carcinogenic substance and it has been linked to skin rashes. Not exactly what you want to be going on your skin. However, you can find it in many cleansers that are designed to be applied to your face and body.

Fragrance and Colors Irritate Your Skin

While perfumes and tints aren't as dangerous as some of the other ingredients mentioned here, you may have a reaction to these. In fact, some women find themselves with severe skin rashes just from using a body wash with fancy fragrances.

Microbeads and the Environment

Only recently have we realized the impact of products like body washes and exfoliating scrubs on the environment. A large number of exfoliating products contain tiny plastic beads designed to slough off dead skin and stimulate the circulation.

When you rinse your face, those microbeads flush into the waste system, but they're too small to be caught by most filters in the sewage processing plants. That means millions of plastic beads flood into the ocean every day, the perfect size to be gulped down by fish. While you might not be eating your face wash, you actually could be ingesting some of it when you eat fish. That's a scary thought.

It isn't difficult to make your own body scrubs and you probably already have the ingredients in your home. Making your own products guarantees that you'll know exactly what is in your scrubs. There will be no more mystery ingredients that could damage your body and you'll even see better results.

Protect your skin, your world and your wallet by making your very own bath products, like the scrubs found in this book. If you want to avoid all the trouble that the store-bought versions will bring, just head to the kitchen and start making your own bath scrubs.

Incredible Exfoliants Already in Your Kitchen

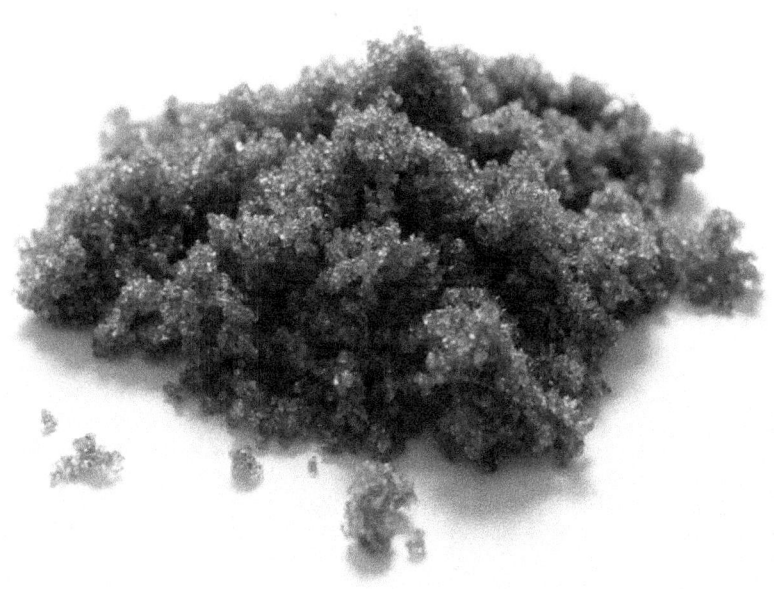

Did you know that your kitchen already contains pretty much everything you need to whip up a great body scrub? Your pantry is the key to glowing skin. While some scrubs require more exotic ingredients, you should be able to create a delightful body product right now if you want to.

Each of the recipes in this chapter are simple enough to whip up, but the real appeal is the complete lack of shopping necessary. You probably have everything you need right now.

Chocolate Body Scrub

Who doesn't love chocolate? This body scrub incorporates coconut oil to moisturize and sugar to exfoliate dead skin. The cocoa stimulates blood flow and makes the whole thing smell wonderful.

¼ cup cocoa

1 cup brown sugar

½ cup coconut oil

Mix the sugar and cocoa thoroughly before adding the coconut oil. Combine well and use immediately or store for up to a week in an airtight container.

Citrus Oatmeal Scrub

This simple recipe gives you a very light and easy scrub. The grapefruit juice will rejuvenate your skin and give you a healthy glow, while the oatmeal exfoliates.

1 grapefruit

2 tablespoons quick oats

Peel the grapefruit and blend the pulp in the blender. Mix in the oatmeal to form a paste and rub it all over your body. You may need to add more oatmeal or a little water to get the right consistency.

Baking Soda Cleansing Scrub

Baking soda is a good gentle exfoliant. It works well for oily skin and is a natural disinfectant with both honey and baking soda. The milk will leave your skin smooth and silky.

¼ cup baking soda

1 tablespoon honey

1 tablespoon milk

Mix the baking soda, honey and milk to make a thick paste and use it immediately.

Zesty Citrus Scrub

The salt and citrus zest in this scrub will help rid you of dead skin cells while giving you a nice little burst of brightness. Your skin will positively glow after your shower.

½ cup olive oil

½ cup salt

1 tablespoon lemon or orange zest

Mix the ingredients until they are well combined. Use the scrub right away.

Simple Salt and Oil Bath Rub

This is one of the simplest ways to rid yourself of dead skin. Everyone has olive oil and salt in their kitchen, so put them to good use!

¼ cup olive oil

½ cup table salt

Mix the two ingredients in a dish until you have a thick paste. Use the mixture immediately.

Pineapple Sugar Scrub

Pineapple is a source of bromelain, which dissolves dead skin right off your body. This could easily be a smoothie, if you were so inclined. The sugar works as an exfoliant to get rid of dead cells while the pineapple dissolves the connections to enable removal.

1 cup fresh pineapple, chopped

¼ cup sugar

Blend the pineapple in the blender until smooth. If it is too liquid, you may want to drain the pineapple slightly. Stir in the salt and use immediately.

Ultimate Sweetness Scrub

This super sweet body scrub is totally edible, but you should probably stick to rubbing it on your body. The honey works as a natural antibiotic and helps rid the skin of bacteria, while the sugar eliminates the upper layer of the dermis. The oil moisturizes and keeps you smelling wonderful.

2 tablespoons raw honey

3 tablespoons olive oil

½ cup brown sugar

Mix the ingredients thoroughly before using. It's a good idea to try this scrub in the shower, since it can be a little sticky. Keep any extra in an airtight container for up to four weeks.

Spiced Latte Scrub

If you enjoy the aroma of a holiday spiced latte, you'll love this scrub. It's so good, you'll be tempted to eat it. Use it on your body, though, for the best results. The coffee helps reduce cellulite, stimulate circulation and it even works as an exfoliant.

1 cup brown sugar

2 tablespoons coffee grounds

2 tablespoons pumpkin pie spice

1 teaspoon cinnamon

¾ cups olive coconut oil

Mix the dry ingredients well and add the oil. Stir until smooth and use immediately.

Lemon Sugar Scrub

The honey and lemon in this recipe both work to disinfect surfaces, which makes them ideal for use with acne. The olive oil will help keep skin soft while dead skin gets the boot from the sugar.

1 tablespoon honey

1 tablespoon oil

¼ tablespoon fresh lemon juice

½ cup Brown sugar

Mix everything until well combined. Use immediately or store in an airtight container for up to a month.

Vanilla Sugar Cookie Scrub

You'll swear you're rubbing sugar cookie dough on your skin with this deliciously scented mixture. The vanilla seeds help exfoliate, but most of this job is done by the sugar.

½ cup brown sugar

1 vanilla bean OR 1 teaspoon vanilla extract

3 tablespoons coconut oil

2 drops lemon essential oil

Mix the coconut oil and lemon essential oil before adding to the sugar. If you are using a vanilla bean, cut the bean in half and scrape the seeds into the scrub. Stir well and use. This may be kept for up to a month in an airtight container.

Cucumber Oatmeal Scrub

While the ingredients in this scrub might seem familiar, you will be using them in a rather unique way. This is a great soothing mixture. You should never apply a scrub to damaged or sunburned skin, but this is great for slightly irritated areas. It's cooling and healing.

½ cup peeled cucumber, chopped

2 tablespoons plain yogurt

2 tablespoons oatmeal

2 tablespoons almond oil

In a blender, puree the cucumber. Add the remaining ingredients and blend to create a smooth paste. Use this mixture immediate and discard any leftovers.

Use These Super Moisturizing Scrubs to Keep Your Skin Soft

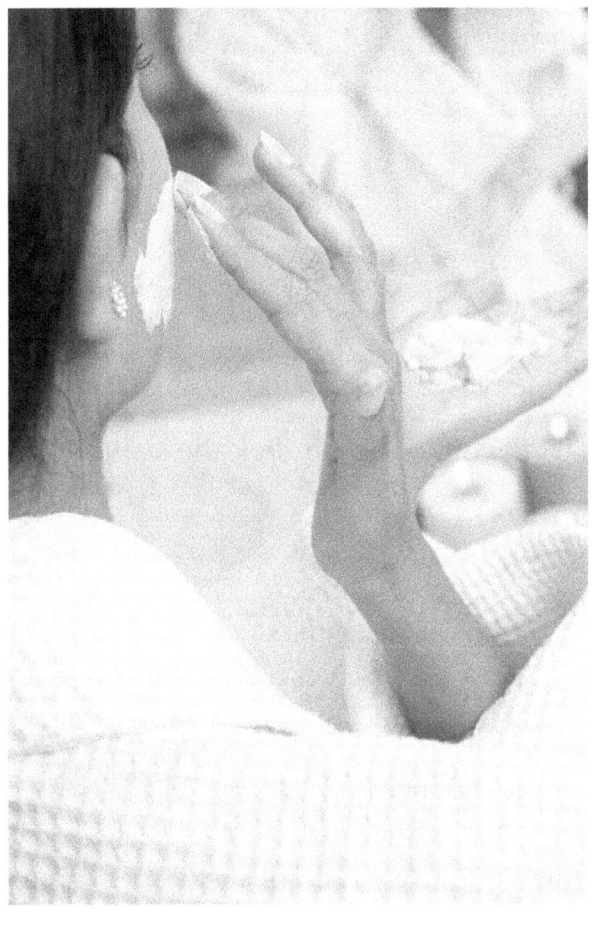

Dry skin can be itchy and uncomfortable. You can skip the moisturizer after exfoliation if you use these super moisturizing scrubs. Each of these recipes features a particular moisturizing ingredient, but getting rid of dried skin will allow it to work even more effectively. Essentially, these scrubs are dual purpose.

To make a hydrating scrub, use oils like almond oil or olive oil, or a moisturizing substance like avocado, banana or shea butter. Combined with an exfoliating ingredient such as salt, sugar or coffee grounds, these ingredients smooth your skin and keep it moisturized at the same time.

Super Soft Coconut Oil Scrub

This scrub will leave your skin silky soft, but it also smells wonderful. The coconut oil will lock the scent of vanilla in and you'll smell of baked goods all day.

1 cup coconut oil

1 cup brown sugar

1 teaspoon vanilla essence

Mix all ingredients until well combined. Keep in an airtight container for up to two weeks.

Banana Split Scrub

Bananas are very good for your face. They work as moisturizers and go well with many other exfoliant ingredients. This is the perfect recipe if you want to avoid using much oil on your skin.

1 overripe banana, mashed

4 tablespoons sugar

1 teaspoon olive oil

Mash the banana with the sugar and oil to get a great scrubbing paste. Use it immediately.

Brown Sugar and Shea Butter Scrub

Brown sugar lends a pleasant scent to this scrub while rubbing away dead cells. The shea butter and oils make it a super moisturizing mixture, too.

½ cup brown sugar

½ cup shea butter

¼ cup coconut oil

Warm the shea butter in a double boiler and beat with a hand mixer until fluffy. Gradually drizzle in the coconut oil while beating until the oil is completely integrated. Stir in the sugar and use immediately or save for up to two weeks in an airtight container.

Papaya Sugar Scrub

In this fruit filled mixture, the sugar scrubs while the oils sooth the skin and help moisturize it. The papaya moisturizes and eliminates dead skin and nourishes the new skin cells.

½ cup sugar

3 tablespoons almond oil

3 tablespoons coconut oil

½ cup fresh papaya

Blend the papaya in the blender until smooth. Stir in the oils until well mixed, then add the sugar. Use the scrub immediately.

Avocado Oatmeal Scrub

Oatmeal is a gentle exfoliant in this mixture, while the avocado and olive oil keep skin smooth and hydrated.

1 avocado

¼ cup oatmeal

1 tablespoon olive oil

Mash the avocado with a fork until it is mostly pureed. Mix the oatmeal and oil into the scrub and use immediately.

Fruity Sugar Scrub

Tasty fruits combine forces to moisturize your skin in this delightful body rub. The papaya and pineapple work to eliminate the dead layer of skin while bananas and oil keep the moisture locked in. The sugar helps scrub away excess cells.

1 overripe banana

½ cup pineapple

½ cup papaya

3 tablespoons coconut oil

½ cup sugar

Blend the fruit in the blender until smooth. Mix in the sugar and oil and use immediately.

Whipped Shea Butter and Almond Scrub

The almond meal in this recipe is a wonderfully gentle exfoliant for your entire body. If you don't want to grind your own meal, you can usually find it in health food stores. The shea butter and almond oil help keep your skin hydrated.

1 cup shea butter

2 tablespoons almond oil

1 cup almonds

Chop the almonds in a grinder or food processor until a fine meal is formed.

In another bowl, beat the shea butter with a hand mixer until it is creamy and fluffy. Drizzle in the avocado oil and vanilla essence and beat until incorporated completely.

Stir in the almond meal and use or store in an airtight container for up to two weeks.

Honey Yogurt Moisturizing Scrub

Yogurt is a good humidifying ingredient to include in your scrubs. It also works to exfoliate, as does honey. Honey prevents skin infections and is particularly good for acne. This scrub does not contain oil and is ideal for those with oily skin.

½ cup plain Greek yogurt

2 tablespoons honey

1 teaspoon cinnamon

2 tablespoons sugar

Mix all the ingredients together until smooth. Use immediately and discard any leftovers.

Honey Bran Body Rub

Bran is the exfoliating ingredient in this sweet smelling recipe. The honey and oil keep your entire body moisturized and clean.

3 tablespoons sugar

2 tablespoons honey

2 tablespoons oat bran

2 tablespoons coconut oil

½ teaspoon vanilla extract

Mix the ingredients well and use. You can store this mixture for up to 3 weeks in an airtight container.

Honey Papaya Scrub

This is a super moisturizing scrub that will benefit you if you need a very strong moisturizer. The honey and papaya both help lock in water and exfoliate at the same time.

½ cup sugar

½ cup papaya, chopped

2 tablespoons honey

3 drops of lemon essential oil

Blend the papaya into a puree in the blender. Stir in the remaining ingredients and use immediately. Discard any leftovers.

The Secret to Fast Energy

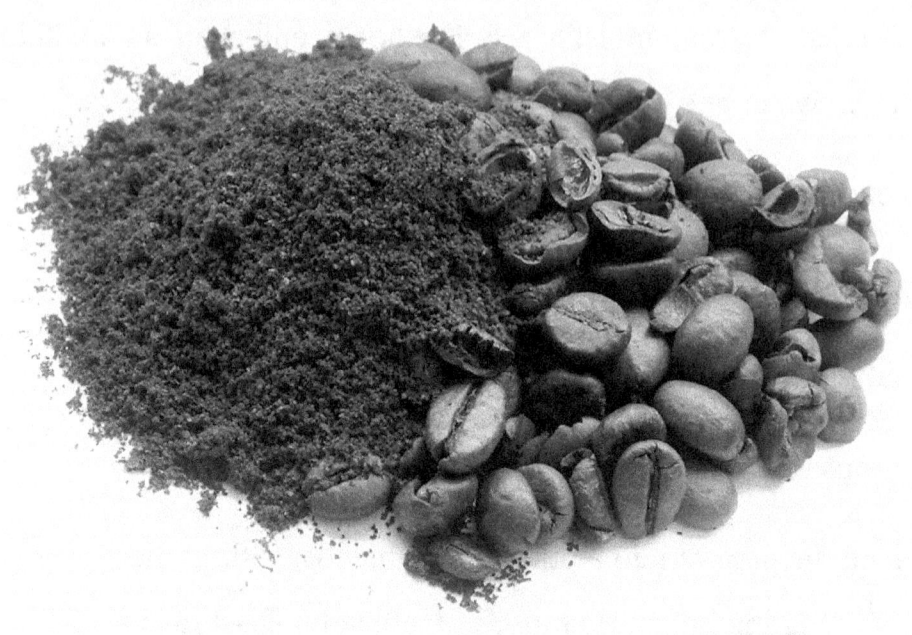

An energizing scrub can do wonders to get your blood flowing. If you're having difficulty waking up before work or need a little more zip before a big test, these body scrubs are perfect. Not only do they strip away dead skin, the scrubs will actually revitalize you!

The ingredients used in these recipes are chosen for their stimulating properties. They will increase circulation wherever you use them and will help banish cellulite. The recipes in this chapter are ideal for those who need a little more energy. They combine skin stimulation with aromatherapy to give you the best results.

Energizing Coffee Scrub

Even if you don't drink coffee, you'll love this scrub that really wakes you up in the morning. It contains two exfoliants, coffee and sugar. The coconut oil moisturizes while the cinnamon and coffee stimulate circulation and help tone the skin.

1 cup ground coffee

1 cup brown sugar

½ cup coconut oil

2 teaspoons ground cinnamon

Mix the dry ingredients and then stir in the coconut oil. It should be in liquid form when you mix it into the scrub. Store the scrub for up to two weeks in a tightly closed container.

Citrus Sugar Blend

The combination of several citrus fruits is what makes this scrub great. It smells heavenly and works very well to exfoliate any area of the body.

1 cup sugar

¼ cup olive oil

3 tablespoons lemon juice

Zest of an orange

Zest of a lime

Zest of a grapefruit

Blend the ingredients until relatively smooth. Use the scrub immediately and discard any leftovers.

Minty Green Tea Scrub

Green tea has many benefits. It is a natural astringent and toner. When you mix it with a bit of mint and some sugar, you have a very potent body scrub.

¼ cup strong brewed green tea

1 cup sugar

2 tablespoons ground almonds

3 drops peppermint essential oils.

Mix all the ingredients in a bowl and use. You can also store it for up to a month in an airtight bag or container.

Rosemary Ginger Energy Scrub

This scrub requires a little more work than most of the recipes shown here, but it is worth it. The rosemary, ginger, and lemon all work to perk up your senses and give you a boost of energy.

1 cup coconut oil

1 cup salt

3 tablespoons rosemary

Zest of 2 lemons

2 tablespoons fresh ginger, minced

Warm the coconut oil over low heat. Add the ginger, rosemary and zest and let it heat for a good ten minutes over low heat. Strain the oil to remove the herbs and cool to room temperature.

Mix the oil into the salt. You can store this for up to a month in a tightly closed container.

Almond Apple Cider Vinegar Rub

Apple cider vinegar is an astringent, so this rub is great for oily skin. It also helps dissolve dead skin. The almonds gently slough off excess cells.

¼ cup almonds

1 tablespoon honey

1 tablespoon apple cider vinegar

8 tablespoons oatmeal

Grind the almonds in a spice grinder or food processor until they are turned to fine meal. Mix with the oatmeal, honey and apple cider vinegar. Use the scrub immediately.

Candy Cane Body Scrub

Sweet treats combine to make this delightful holiday scrub one that will give you a little buzz. The peppermint oil is bound to wake you up and stimulate blood flow, while the oil moisturizes and the sugar sloughs off skin.

2 cups brown sugar

5 drops peppermint oil

½ teaspoon vanilla extract

½ cup olive oil

½ cup almond oil

Mix the oils together and add to the sugar. Stir well and mix in the vanilla. Use the mixture immediately or store in an airtight container for up to four weeks.

Rosemary Basil Scrub

Fresh herbs make this scrub an invigorating one. If you prefer not to use a sweet scented exfoliating mix, then this is a great option.

3 tablespoons salt

2 tablespoons fresh rosemary

2 tablespoons fresh basil

2 tablespoons olive oil

Use a spoon to mash the herbs into the salt until the salt turns green. Add the oil and mix well. Use this scrub immediately and discard any leftovers.

Invigorating Lemon-Lime Scrub

Citrus fruit stimulates circulation and helps give your skin a clean look. It's also useful in reducing oil and dry skin. This recipe uses two aromatic citrus fruits, along with salt, to create a scrub that rejuvenates the body.

2 tablespoons lime juice

2 tablespoons lemon juice

¼ cup salt

Combine the salt with the juices to form a thick paste and use immediately.

Ginger Lemon Scrub

Ginger has been used for centuries to boost the immune system and it is also useful in increasing your circulation. Lemon is a natural astringent and cleanser, as well as an exfoliant.

2 tablespoons lemon juice

½ teaspoon ground ginger

1 tablespoon olive oil

4 tablespoons sugar

Mix the ground ginger and sugar together, then add the oil and lemon juice to form a thick paste. Use immediately.

Peppermint Mocha Scrub

For a real pick-me-up, try this delicious smelling scrub. The peppermint and coffee do a lot to stimulate the senses, but the ingredients also boost the blood flow wherever they are used. Coffee grounds are a nice gentle exfoliant, but the sugar adds a little more scrubbing power.

1 cup brown sugar

5 tablespoons coffee grounds

3 tablespoons coconut oil

1 teaspoon peppermint extract

Mix the sugar and coffee and add the oil gradually until you have a thick paste. Add the extract and mix well. Use or store in a tightly closed container for up to a month.

Basil Lime Salt Scrub

While this may sound more like a marinade than a beauty product, it is very good for your skin and stimulating, as well. The strong scents are not for everyone, however, so you may want to substitute lighter scents if you prefer.

1 cup Epsom salts

½ cup almond oil

6 drops lemon essential oil

3 drops basil essential oil

Mix the essential oils into the almond oil until well blended. Stir the mixture into the Epsom salts. You should have a damp sand consistency. This mixture may be used immediately or stored for up to two months in an airtight container.

Rosemary Lavender Scrub

While lavender is a relaxing herb, rosemary is a stimulant and the two herbs work in harmony in this recipe. The oil and salt moisturize and exfoliate.

1 cup salt

3 tablespoons olive oil

3 tablespoons lavender, minced

3 tablespoons rosemary leaves, minced

Blend the herbs into the salt. Stir in the oil and use the mixture within the next three days. This is a good scrub for your face, as well as the rest of your body.

Tips for Perfect Body Scrubs

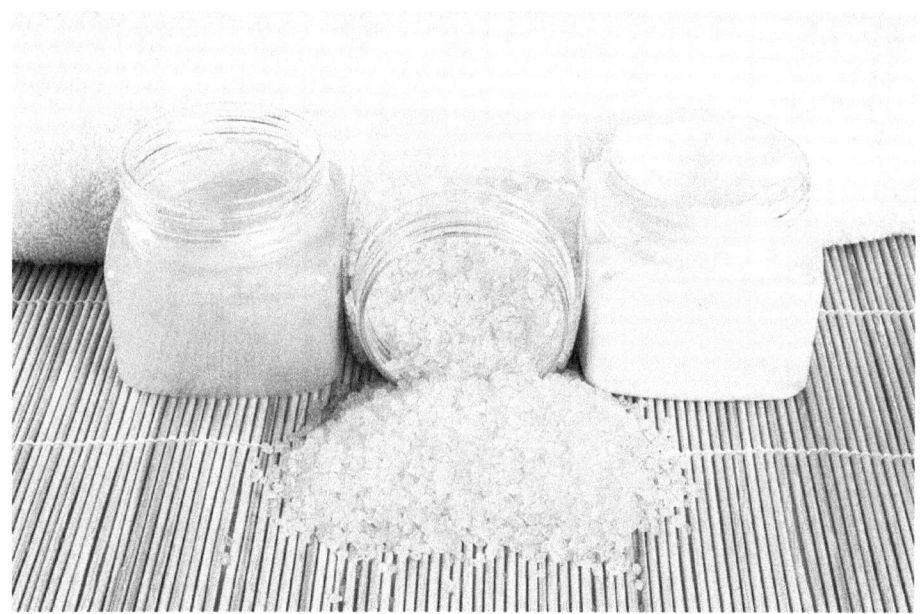

The recipes in this book will stand you in good stead, whether you are trying to regain a healthy, polished look or want to moisturize your dry skin. However, you can also experiment and add your own ingredients to increase how effective your body scrubs are.

Try Aromatherapy

Essential oils are a great addition to any scrub. Choose the oil according to the desired effect. Here are a few of the more common choices:

Calming (ideal for promoting sleep or easing nervous tension)

Lavender

Lemon balm

Chamomile

Stimulating

Lemon

Peppermint

Basil

Rosemary

Spearmint

To get the benefits of the essential oils, you just have to add a couple of drops of any oil to your scrub. It will blend into the other oils and add a unique scent. Don't be afraid to mix scents, too, for even more aromatic punch.

Getting More Use from Your Scrubs

Chances are, you already know how to use a body scrub, but did you know that the best ones are the perishable kind? When you mix up a scrub with your own ingredients, you know they're fresh because they won't last very long.

The best way to use your homemade body scrub is to jump in the shower and to get your entire body wet. Then you can apply the scrub by gently rubbing it over your body in small circles. To get even more from the mixture, try using a pair of exfoliation gloves. These remove extra dry skin, too and work well in combination with the recipes given here.

If you plan to exfoliate your face, you should use very light movements to prevent damage. The skin on your face is more delicate than other areas of your body and may not hold up well to harsher treatments. Mixtures with oatmeal or fruit are good options for facial cleansers.

The exfoliants used in many of these recipes are salt or sugar. These are two ingredients that nearly everyone has in their home. However, you can also use ingredients like citrus zest, ground nuts or even oat bran. The world is full of mildly abrasive ingredients that work well in these homemade beauty products.

Don't Make These 9 Exfoliation Mistakes

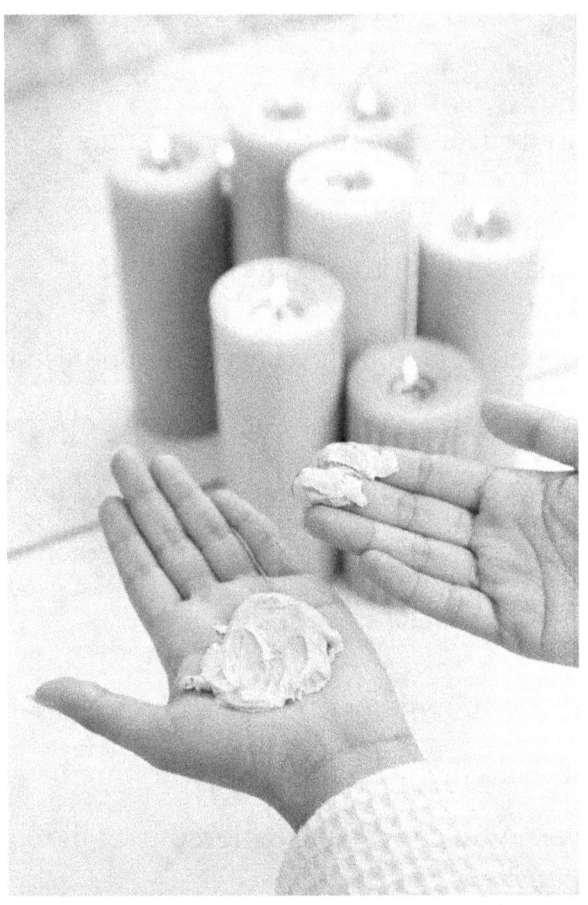

Exfoliating is good for you . . . most of the time. Don't make these mistakes that could ruin your love for scrubs!

Don't :

1. Exfoliate daily. Once you've cleared away the dead skin, it will take a while for the new cells to die off. A common mistake is to use a scrub every day, but this only damages new skin if done too often. Scrubbing once a week is plenty if you have normal skin. Oily skin may be exfoliated twice a week, but keep in mind that even if your face is oily, the rest of your body probably isn't.

2. Use hard particles. Most of the recipes you'll find here use some sort of particle such as sugar or salt to help get rid of the outer layer of dermis. Keep in mind, though, that very hard pieces, like pumice or apricot pits, can actually do more damage to your body. The hard edges cause micro-abrasions which can result in infections and breakouts.

3. Moisturize before exfoliating. Moisturizers are essential if you want to keep your skin well hydrated, but they can also act like glue, plastering the dead cells to your body. You should use your scrub before you add lotion or cream to your skin. This will also allow the moisturizer to really penetrate your skin.

4. Scrub too hard. Again, those little particles in your scrub can cut your skin if you're pushing too hard. While it is called a body scrub, that doesn't mean you should actually scrub it in. Instead, rub the mixture gently in a circular motion to remove dead cells without destroying your skin.

5. Ignore your body. It might be tempting to just exfoliate your face, but this is something that your whole body can benefit from. You'll be glowing from head to toe.

6. Use chemical concoctions. When you make your own body scrubs, you can skip all the nasty additions that seem to pop up in nearly every product on the market. If you're using chemicals on your skin, you're probably getting more than you bargained for.

7. Skip the moisturizer. Exfoliation can be drying to the skin. If you skip the lotion after your exfoliation session, you'll end up with super dry skin that will be even itchier than before. Smooth on a gentle lotion once you've finished with the scrub and rinsed it off. You will notice a big difference.

8. Use a dry scrub. Scrubs should never be used dry. This just increases the chances of being cut and you can ensure that this doesn't happen by using only handmade oil scrubs or adding enough water to a dry scrub to make a paste. This will give a gentler exfoliating action and is less likely to damage your skin.

9. Avoid regular exfoliation. It's important to keep your pores clear and your skin rejuvenated. While exfoliation can be a bad thing if you do it every day, it's also not a good idea to leave it too long. Be sure to treat your skin to an exfoliation at least once a month to keep it clear.

As long as you steer clear of these common mistakes, you can enjoy your regular exfoliation sessions and see some impressive benefits from them.

Conclusion

When body scrubs are so easy to whip up yourself, why would you waste your money on a tiny tub of chemicals and plastics that could ruin your skin? You can vary the ingredients in your scrubs to make sure they suit your needs perfectly and fine tune them to give you precisely the result you want.

Even if you aren't interested in experimenting, try making the recipes given here. They are designed to give specific results and there are enough variations that you should be able to make several of them with the ingredients you have at this very moment in your home.

You can, and should, use a body scrub before you do any kind of skin treatment. If you are planning on doing a henna tattoo, for example, it will last far longer if you remove the dead skin ahead of time. Likewise, you will need to exfoliate before waxing or applying sunless tanning lotion. The end result will be much smoother.

Scrubs can also be helpful in reducing the appearance of cellulite, if you have it. The cottage cheese skin is unpleasant looking, but stimulating the circulation of blood to the area can help reduce the appearance. In fact, anything stimulating, with coffee as one of the ingredients, can help your cellulite look less bumpy.

Full body exfoliation is the best way to look after your skin. Keep your body healthy and free of dull, dead skin that blocks up pores by regularly using a body scrub. It's the best way to spoil yourself!

www.ingramcontent.com/pod-product-compliance
Lightning Source LLC
Chambersburg PA
CBHW070403290526
45790CB00004B/1622